The Abled Little Elephant

SarahJean Harrison

Dedication

Dedicated to Eric Reson and Angela Sanau.

This book serves as a token of my appreciation for their efforts in preserving Kenya's biodiversity for generations to come.

Acknowledgment

In recognition of my husband, David Staples, who embraces continuous learning to overcome challenges posed by his own disability, and for enabling me to pursue both national service and the creation of this book through his unwavering support.

About the Author

Sarah Jean Harrison is a conservationist, a breast cancer survivor, and a Foreign Service Officer at the United States Agency for International Development. Her diverse portfolio of assignments includes Iraq, the Democratic Republic of the Congo, Haiti, Kenya, Israel, and Washington, DC. With a keen focus on environmental conservation, she draws inspiration from her extensive travels and the meaningful connections she forges abroad.

The views expressed in this book are solely the opinions of the author and do not represent those of the U.S. Government.

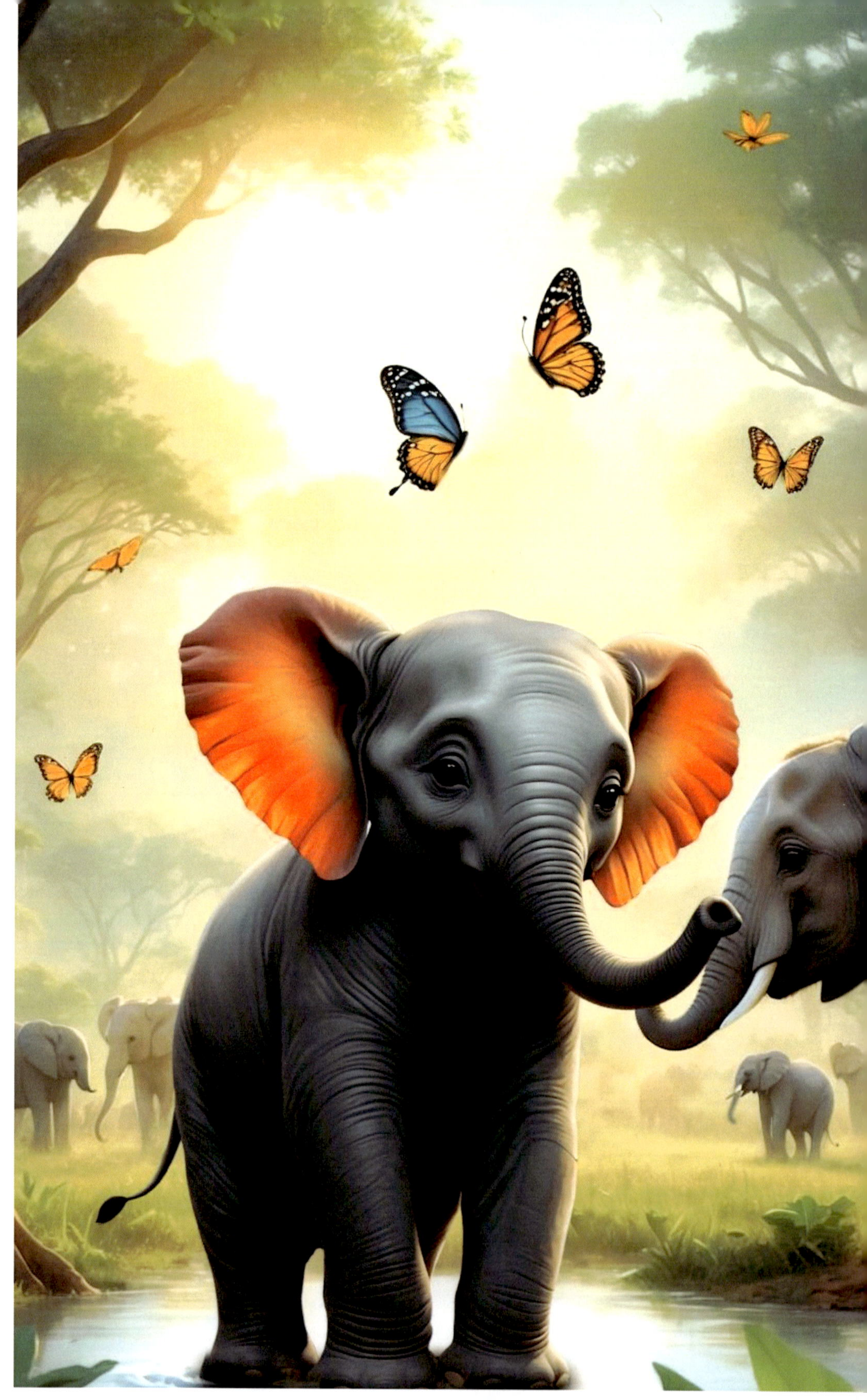

In Southern Kenya lies a lush savannah, where the golden sun kisses the earth, and the tall grasses dance in the breeze. There lived a young elephant named Esinka.

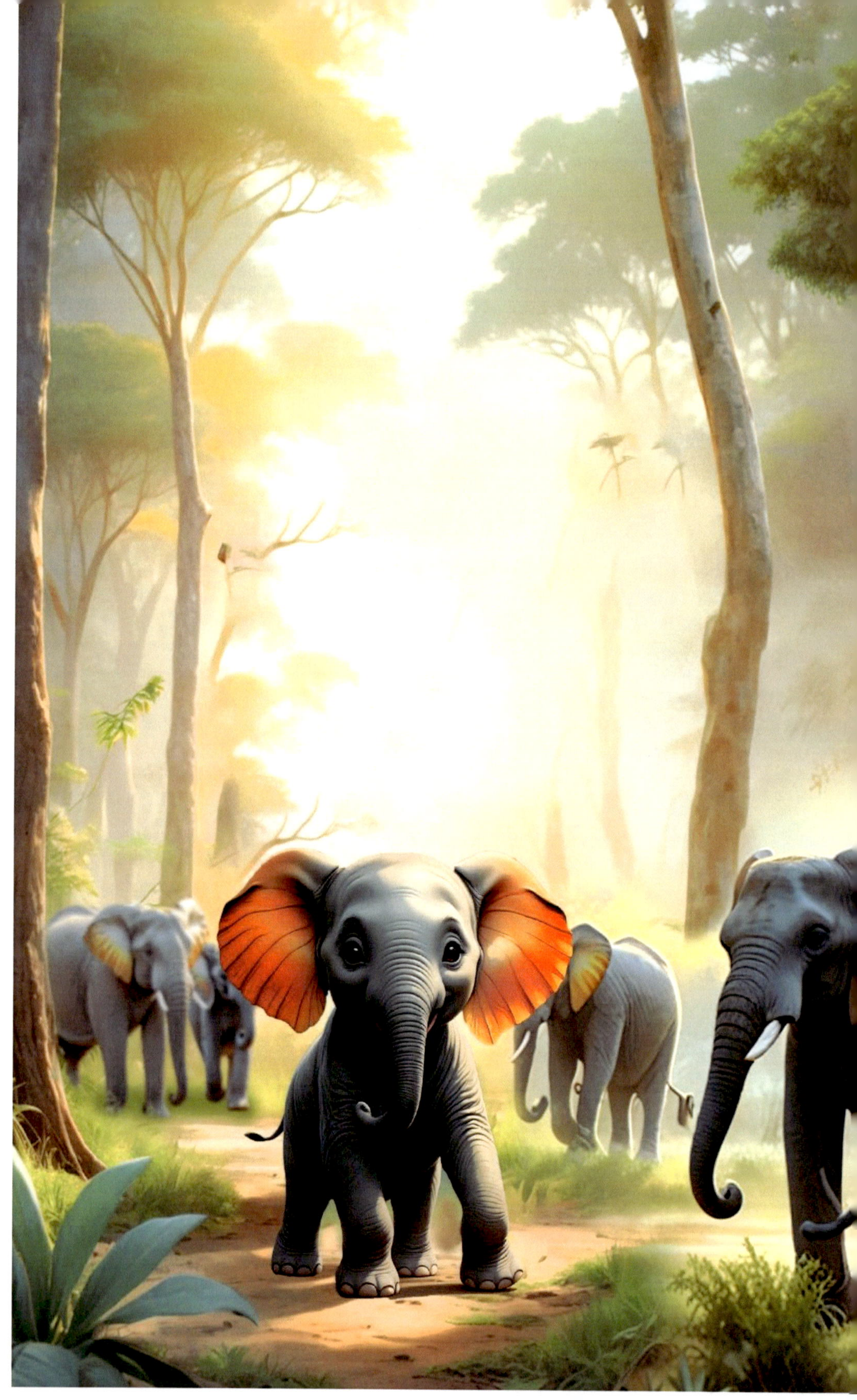

With his curious eyes and playful spirit, Esinka roamed the land alongside his family, exploring the wonders of their wild home.

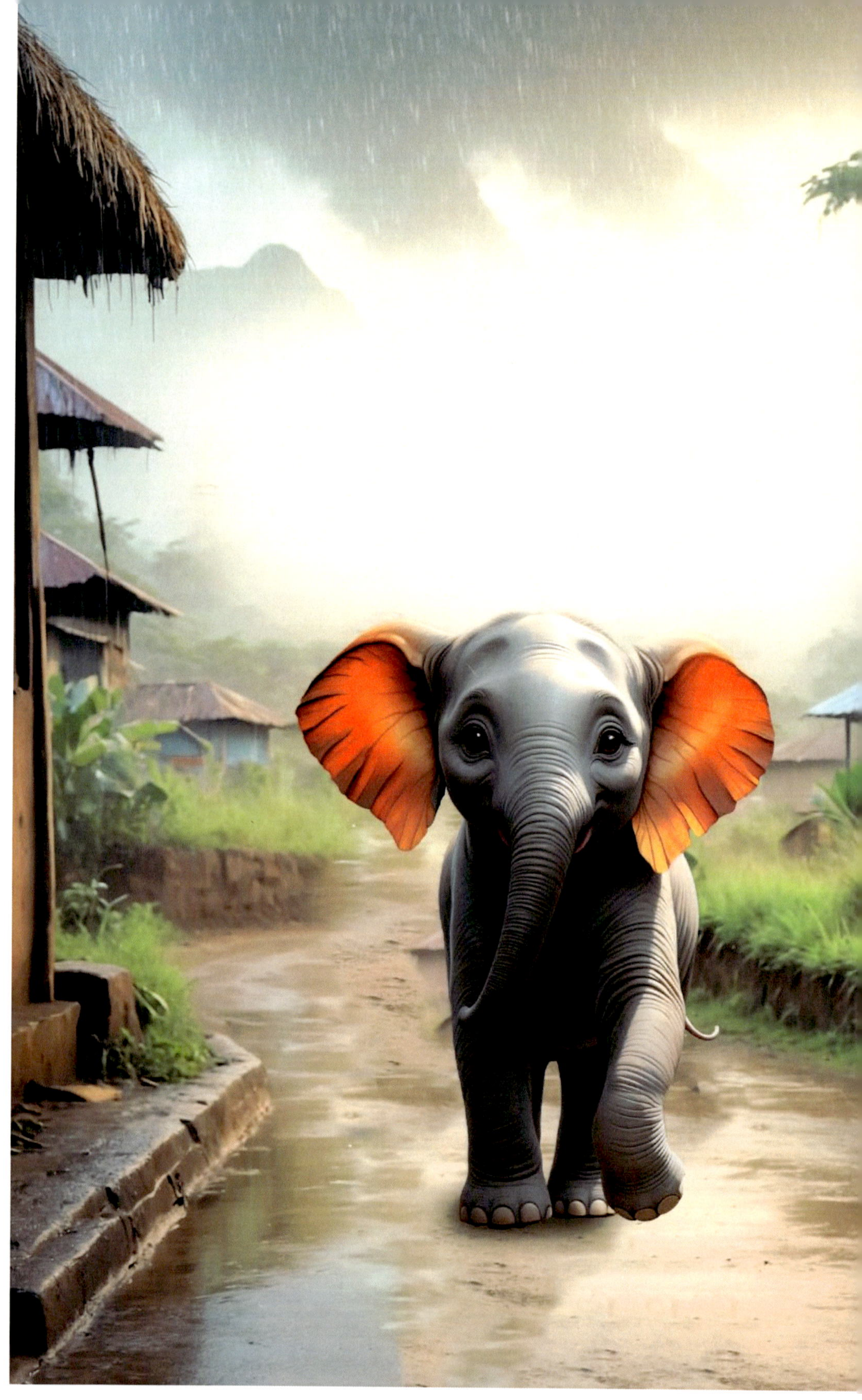

One rainy morning, as Esinka reached near the edge of the Maasai village, his curiosity made him wander.

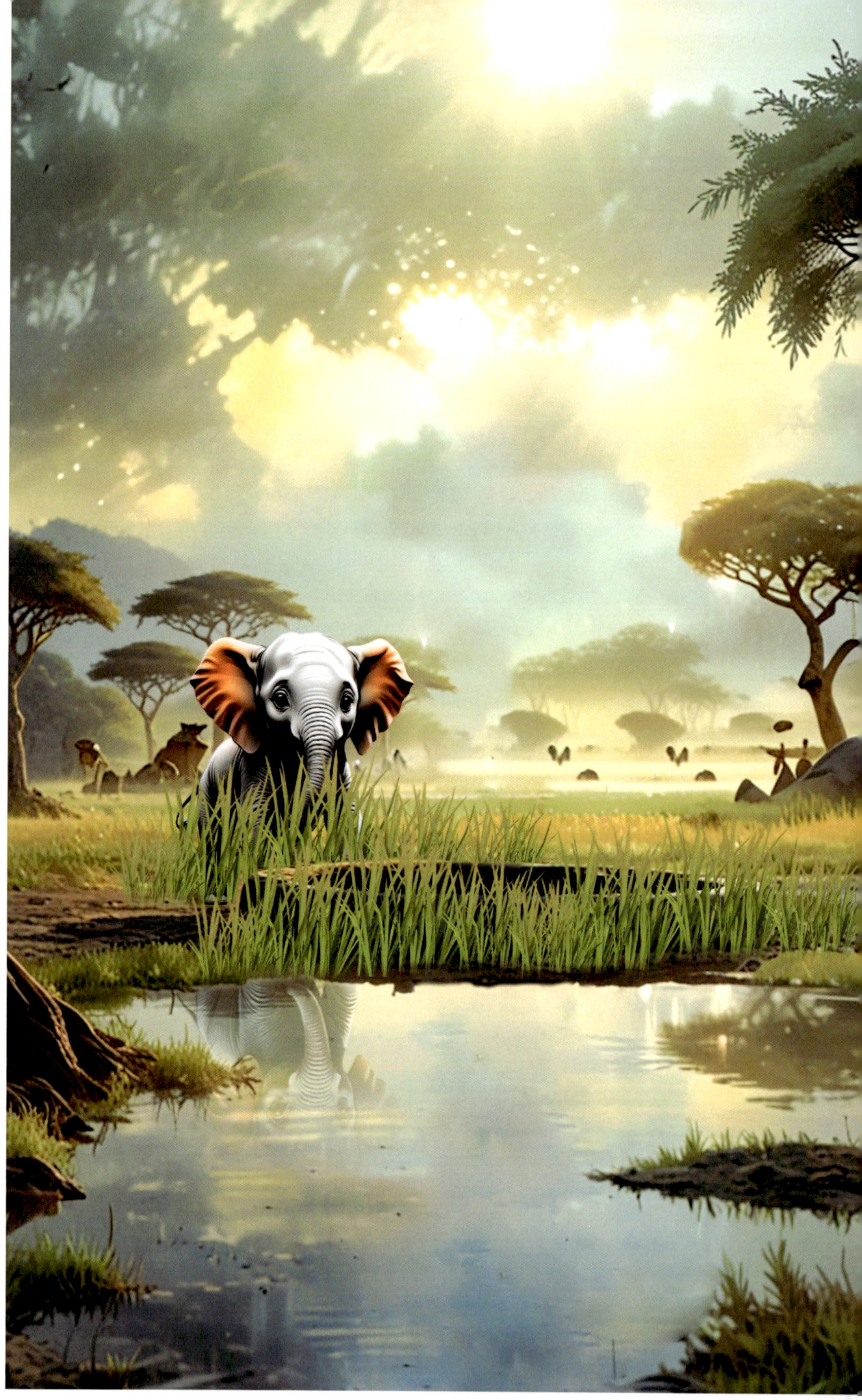

Suddenly he came upon an open well

with tall grasses.

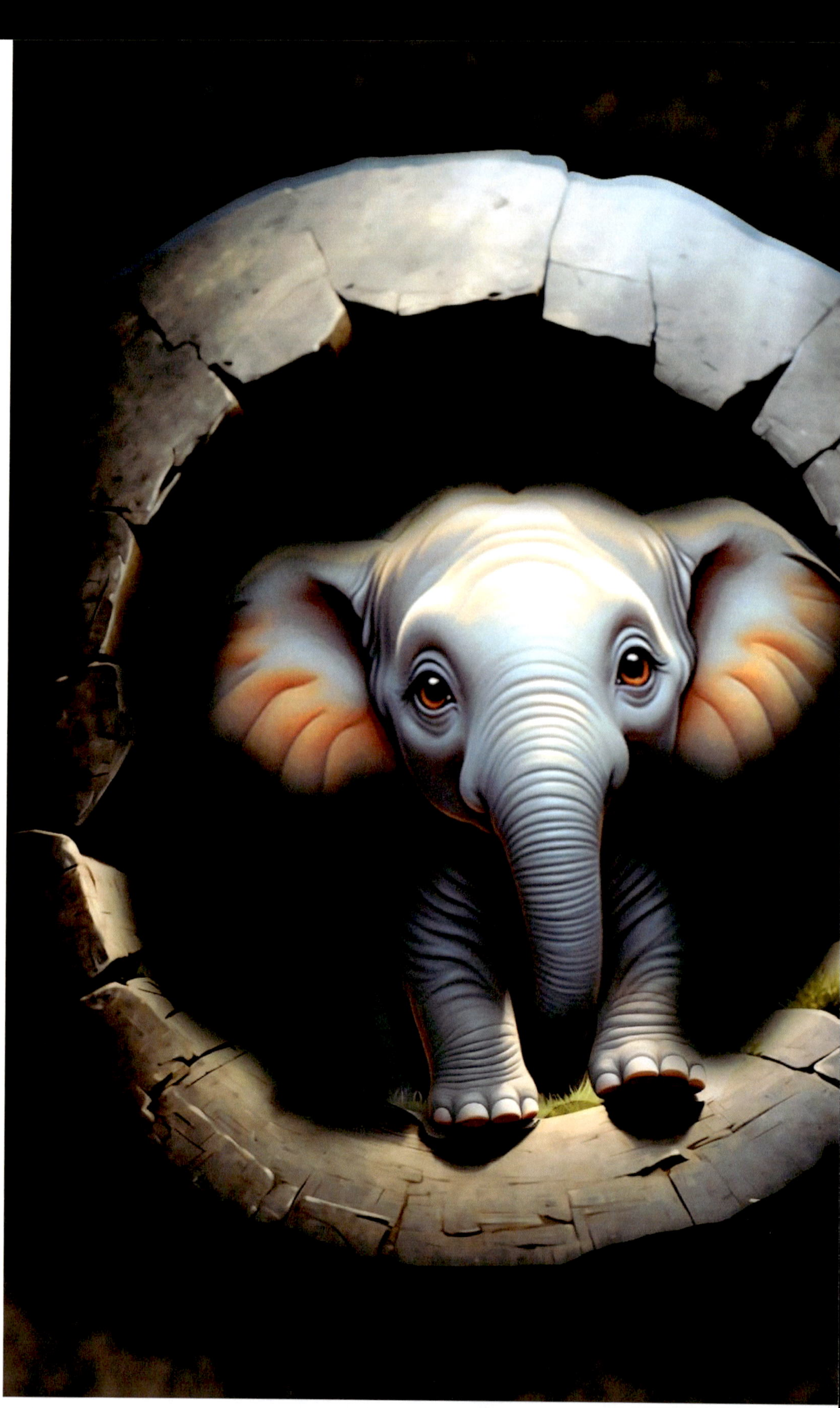

Before he could react, he tumbled into the darkness below, his cries echoing through the air.

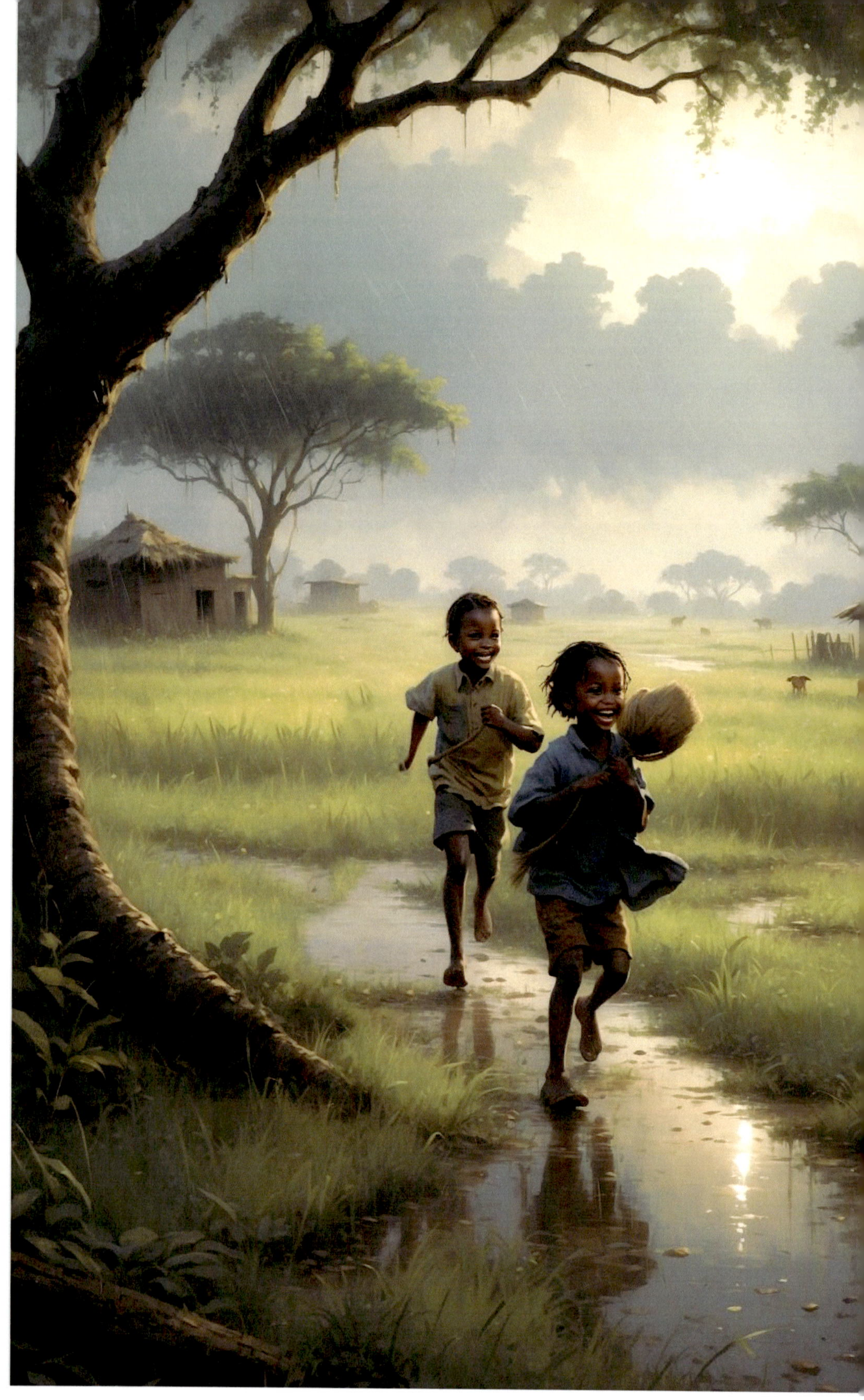

As fate would have it, Angela and Eric,

two adventurous children from the

village, were playing nearby.

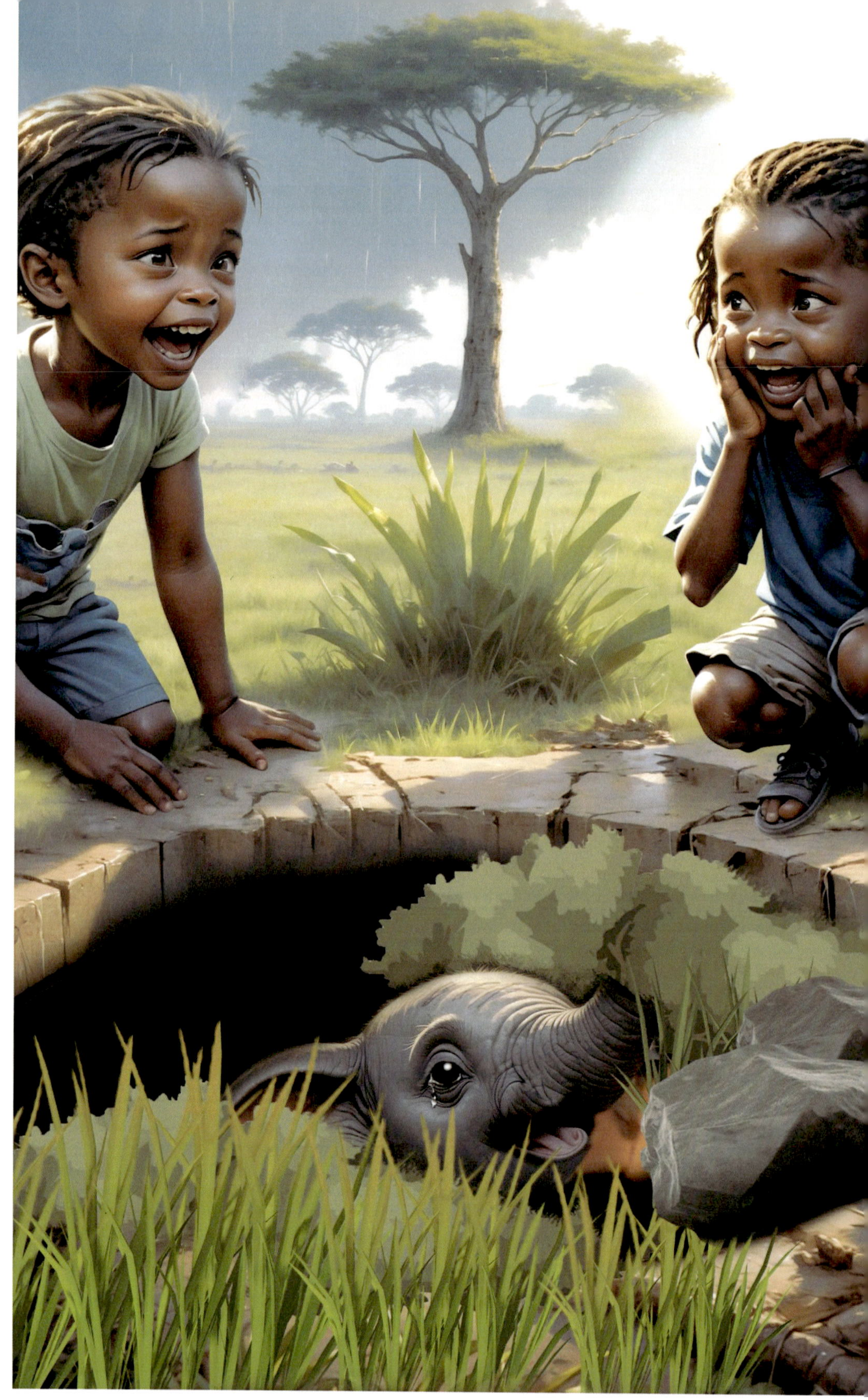

Startled by Esinka cries, they followed

the sounds, found the well, and looked

inside. With horror, they saw Esinka

trapped at the bottom, his trunk caught

in debris.

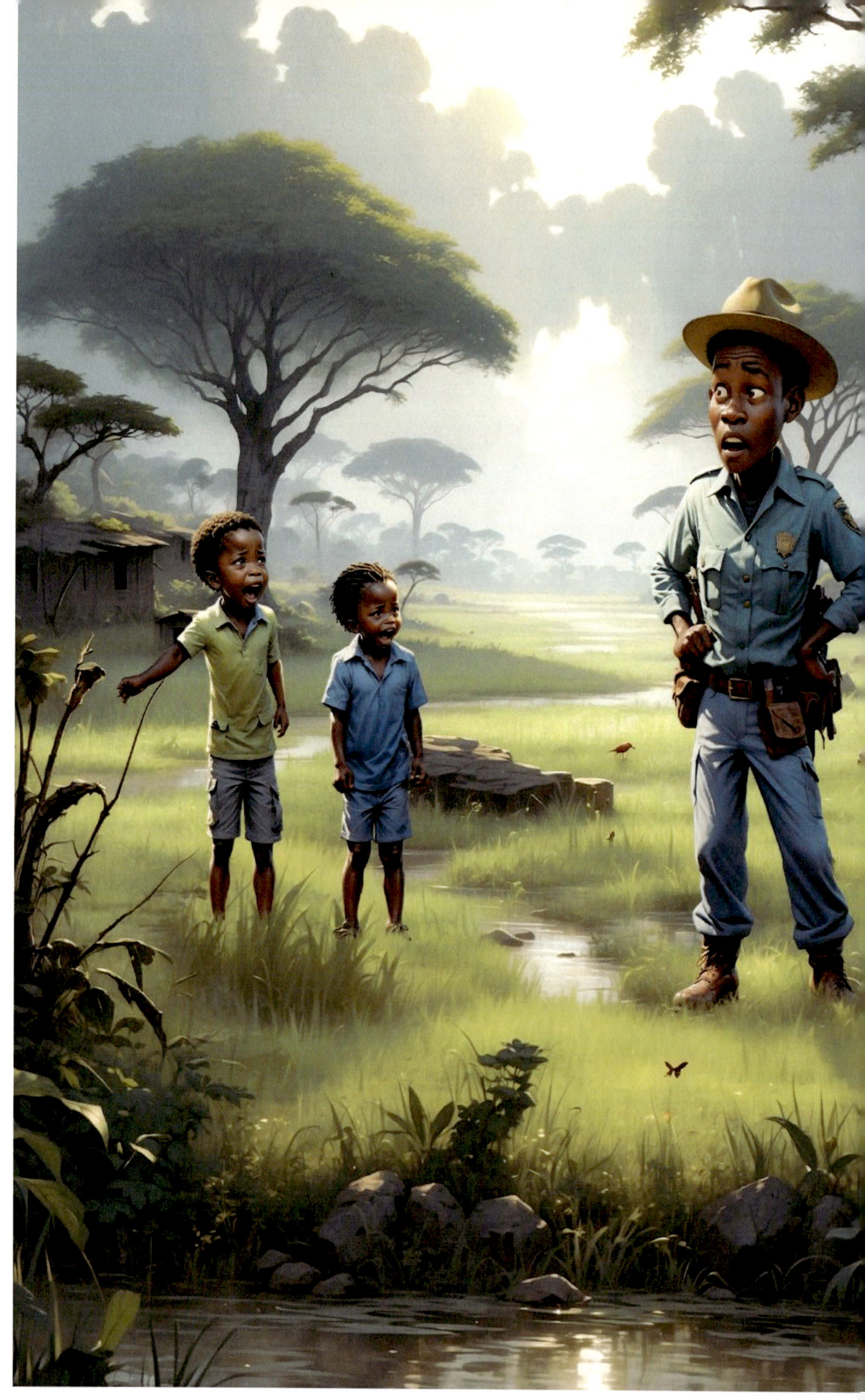

Without hesitation, Angela and Eric

dashed to the nearby elephant

sanctuary, where guards stood watch

over the gentle giants.

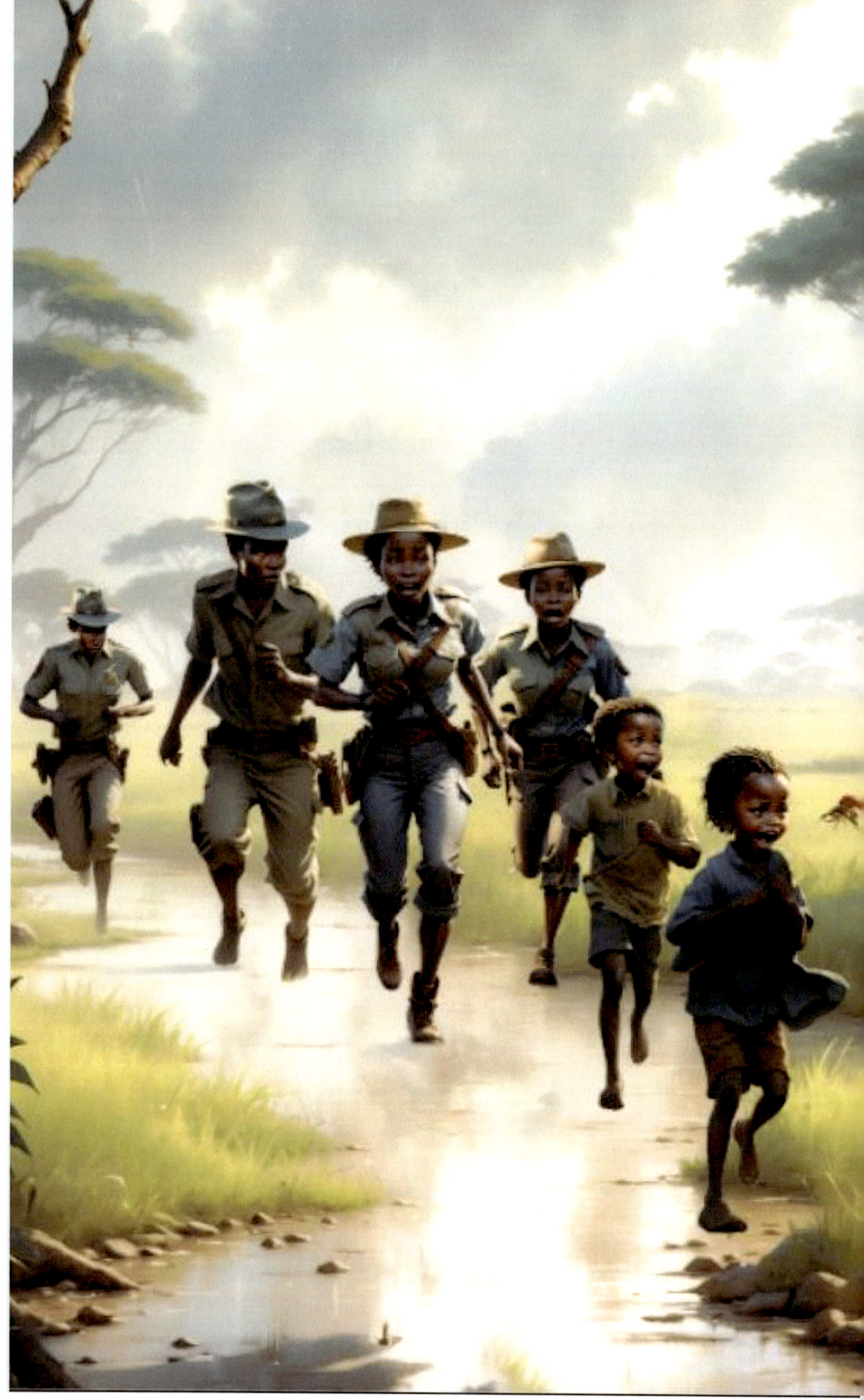

Guided by Angela and Eric, they raced

back to the well, their hearts pounding

with fear and hope.

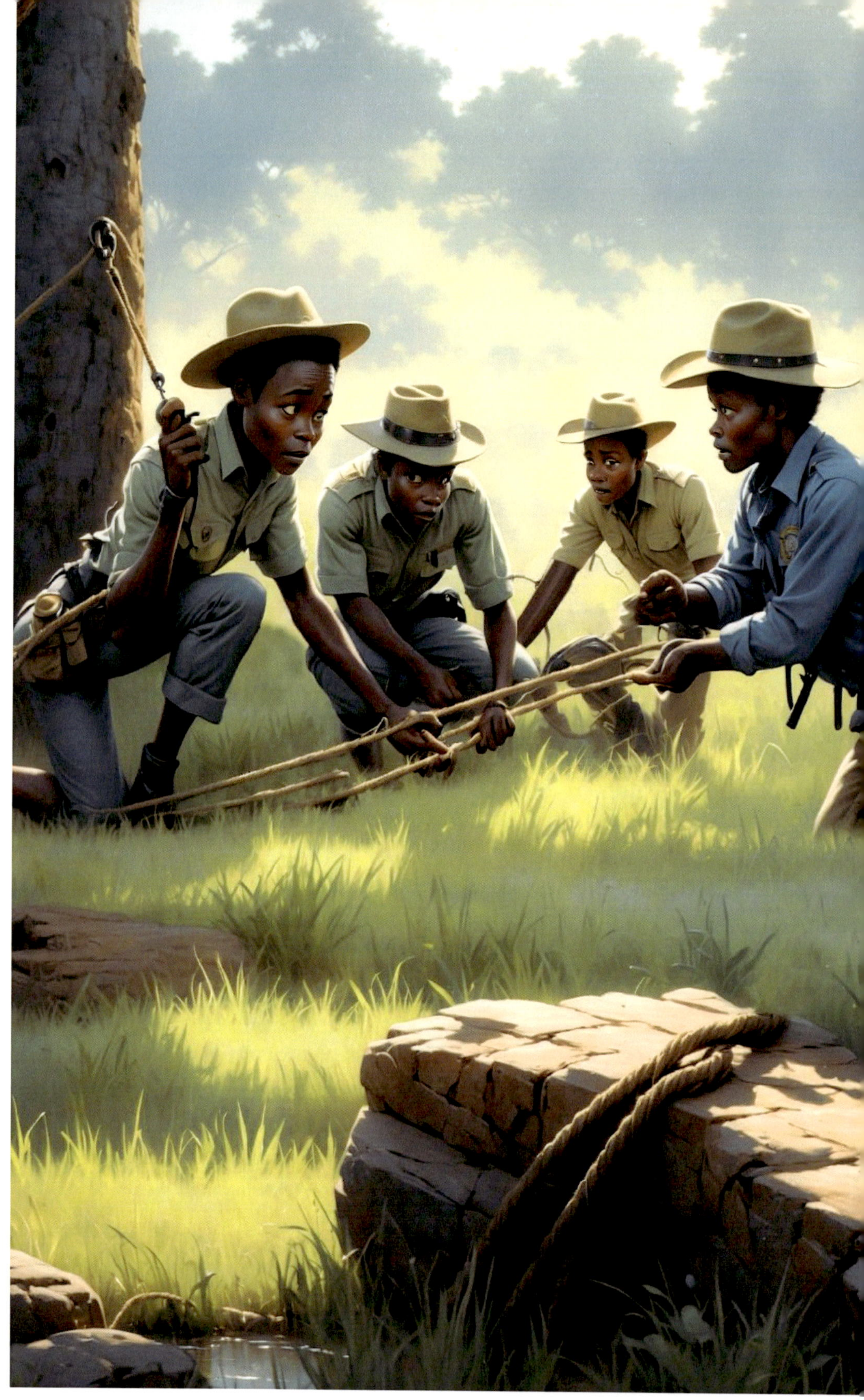

With urgency in their hearts, the

guards sprang into action. They

gathered ropes and pulleys, determined

to rescue Esinka.

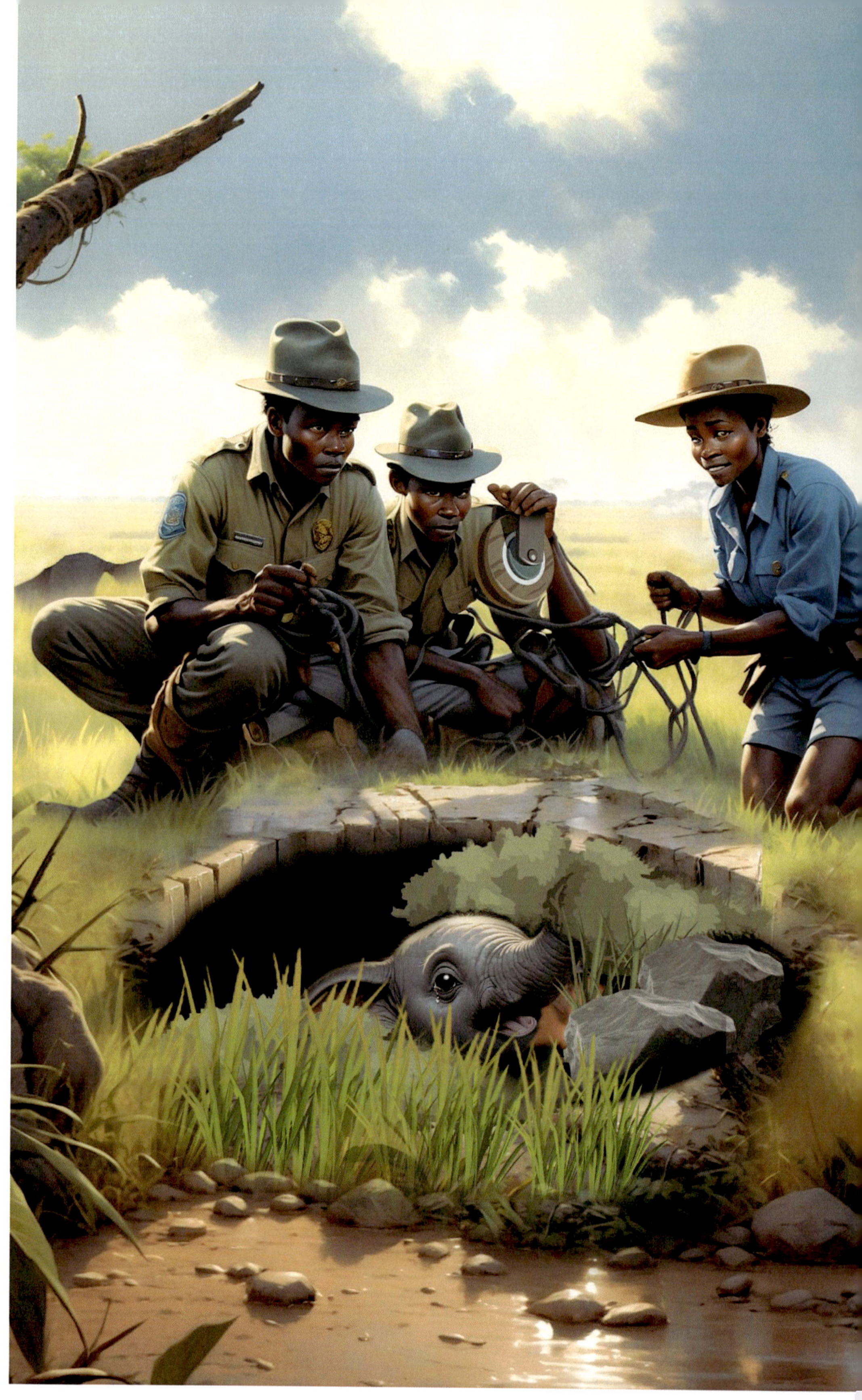

With skill and precision, the guards

lowered themselves into the well,

inching closer to Esinka with each

passing moment. Despite his fear and

pain, Esinka remained remarkably

calm, trusting that the humans wanted

to help him.

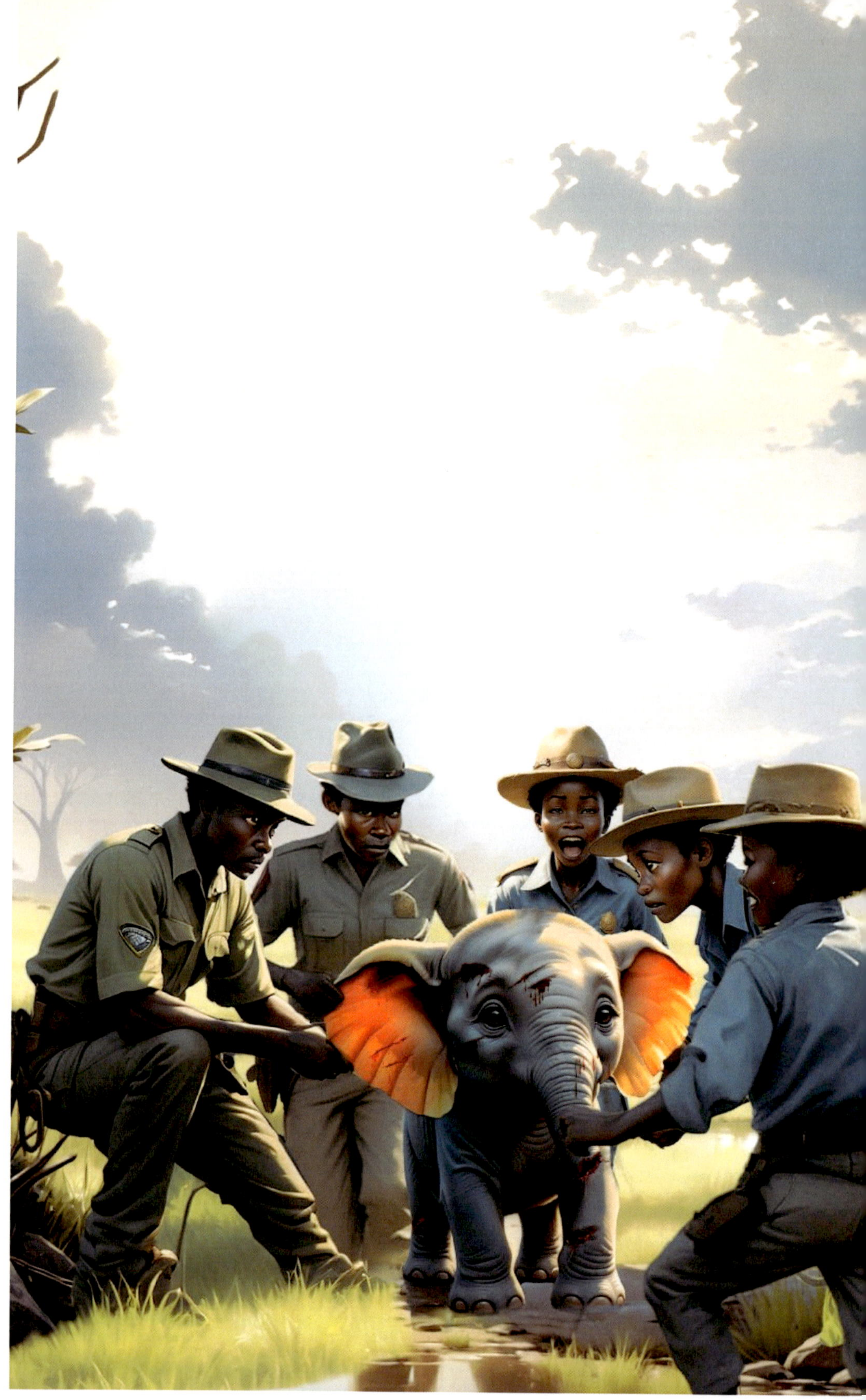

As the sun dipped below the horizon,

casting long shadows across the land,

the guards finally were able to free him

from the debris, lifting him to safety

with tears of relief in their eyes.

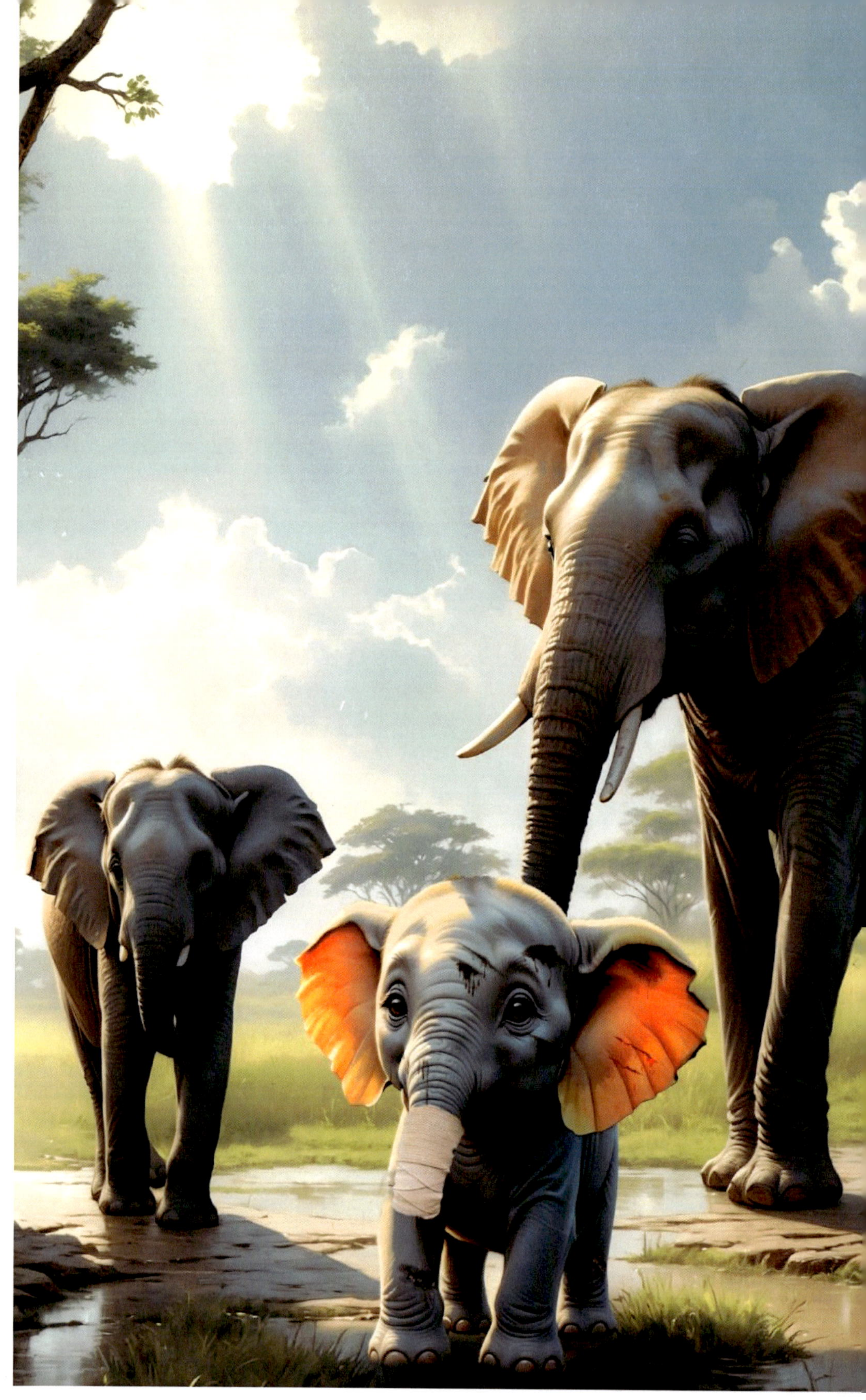

Sadly, Esinka's trunk was cut off in the fall, but with the help of the guards, he was brought to the sanctuary.

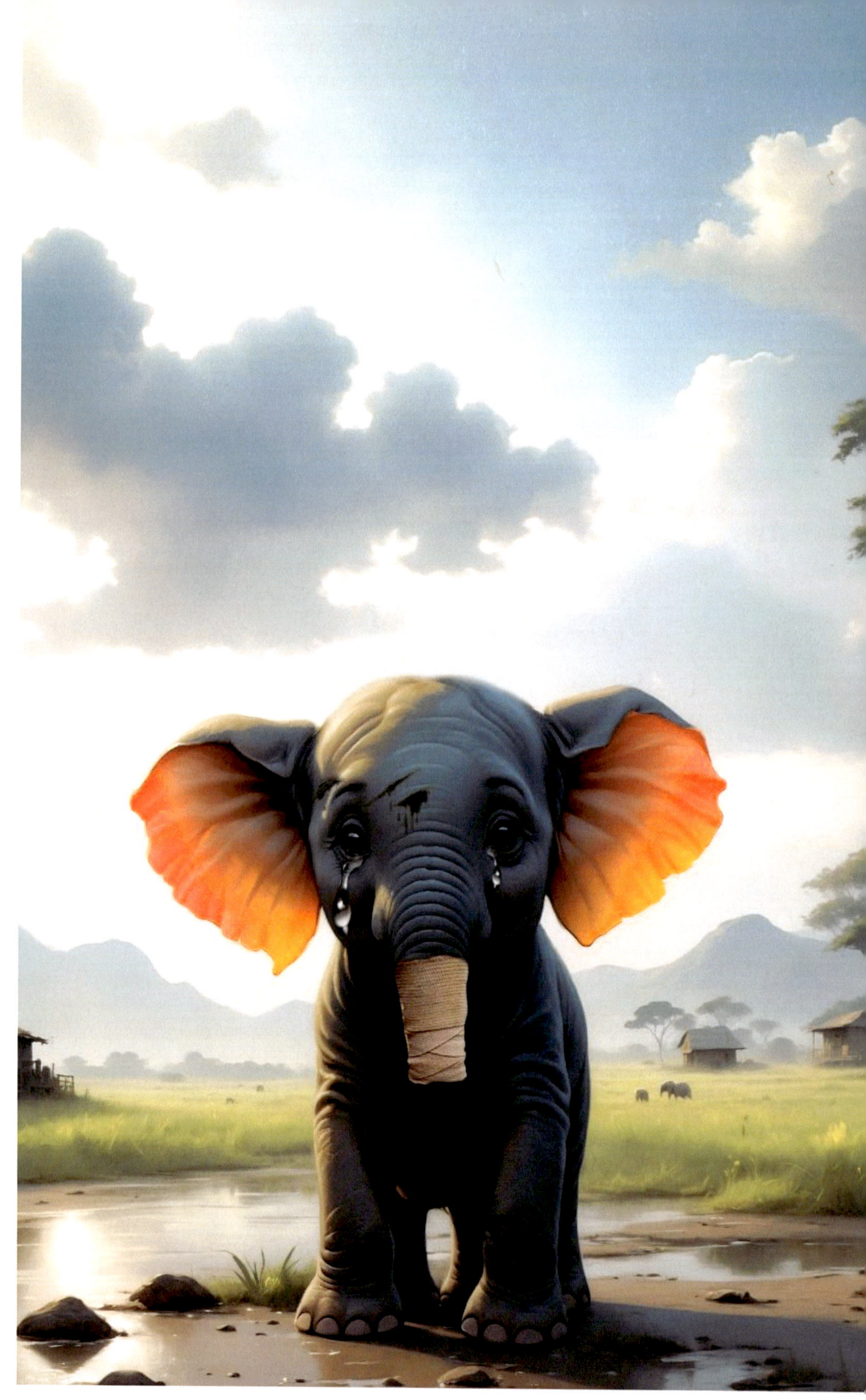

At first, Esinka felt lost and alone.

Although he was happy to be safe, he

was still sad about missing his trunk.

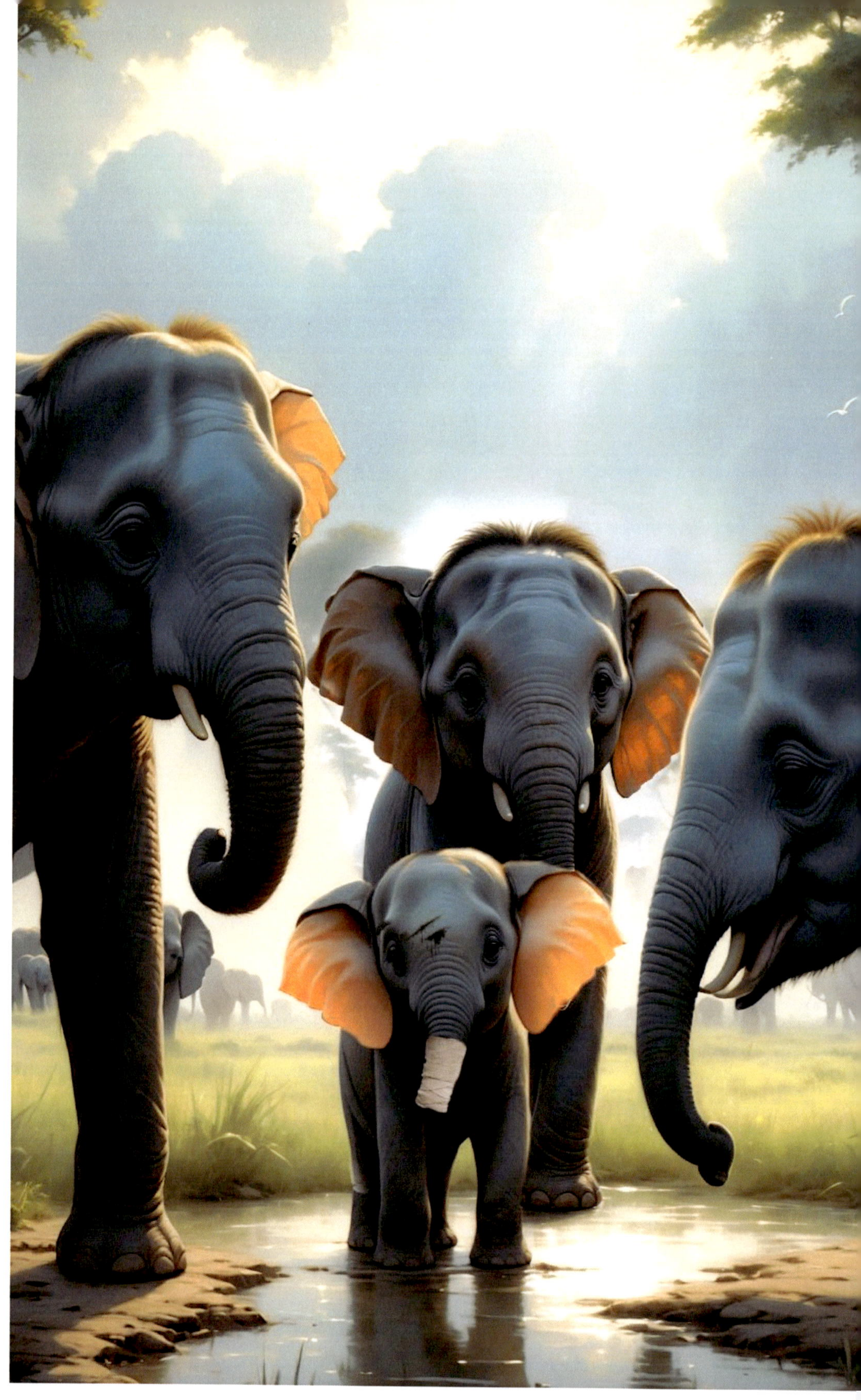

Some of the elephants whispered and pointed at him, making him feel even more different. Some elephants even teased Esinka, calling him names and laughing at the way he looks. Esinka felt hurt and alone, wishing he could hide away from the unkind words.

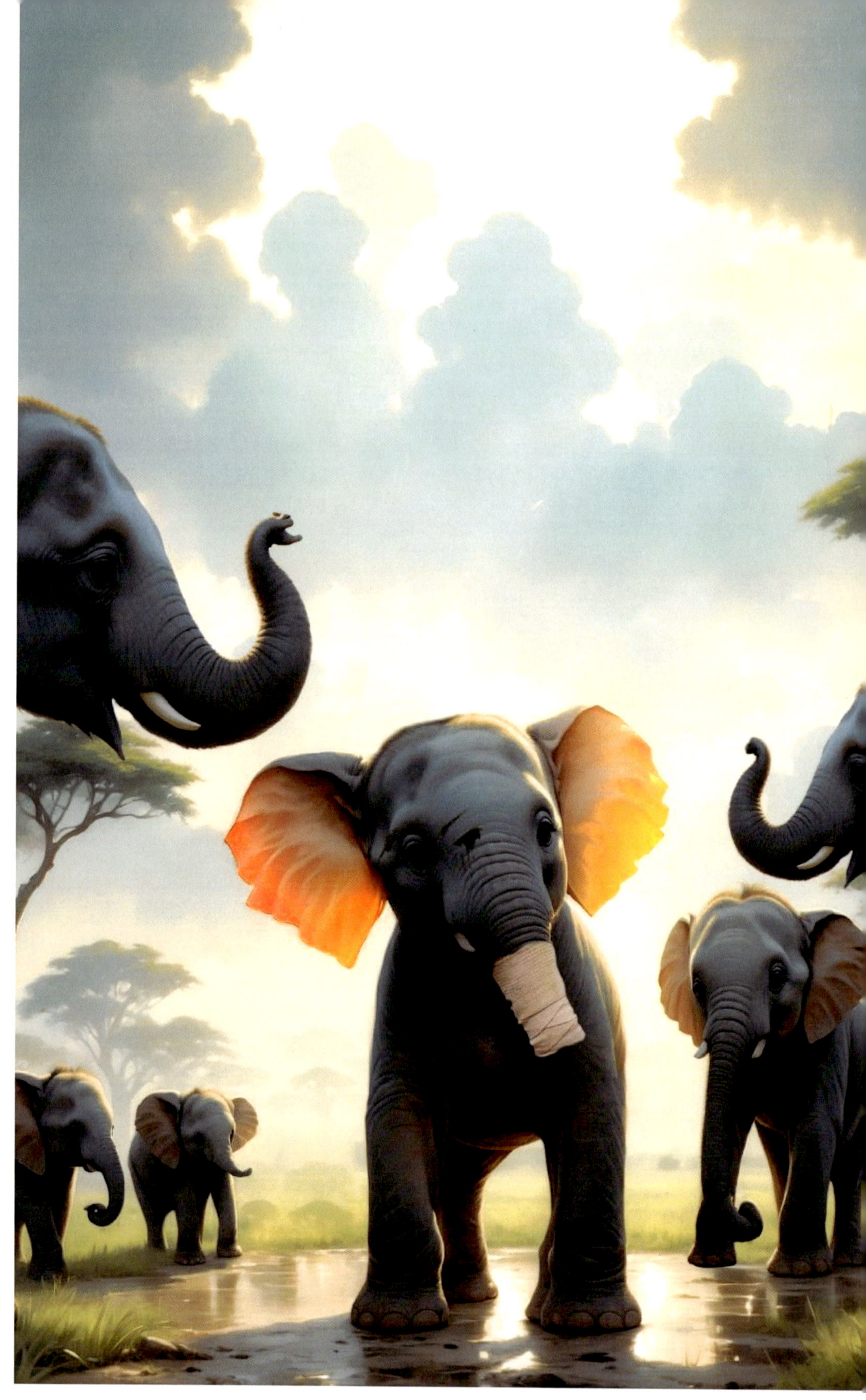

But not all the elephants were unkind.

Some stood up for Esinka, offering him

comfort and friendship. They reminded

him that he was still a strong elephant,

no matter what happened to his trunk.

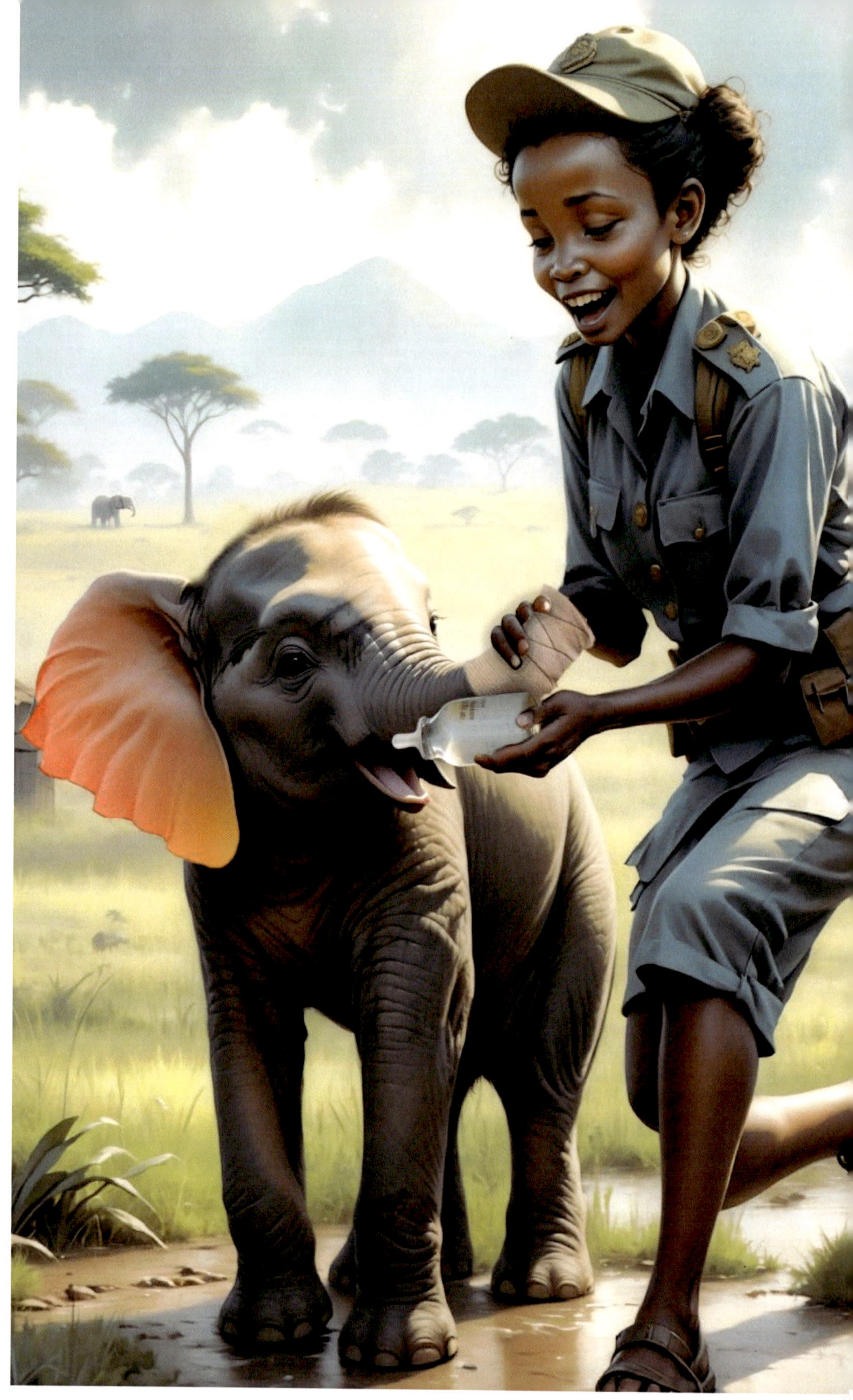

As Esinka healed from his wounds, the guards made sure he remained healthy by feeding him milk from a bottle. He watched his new friends play in the sanctuary and he wanted to be just like them.

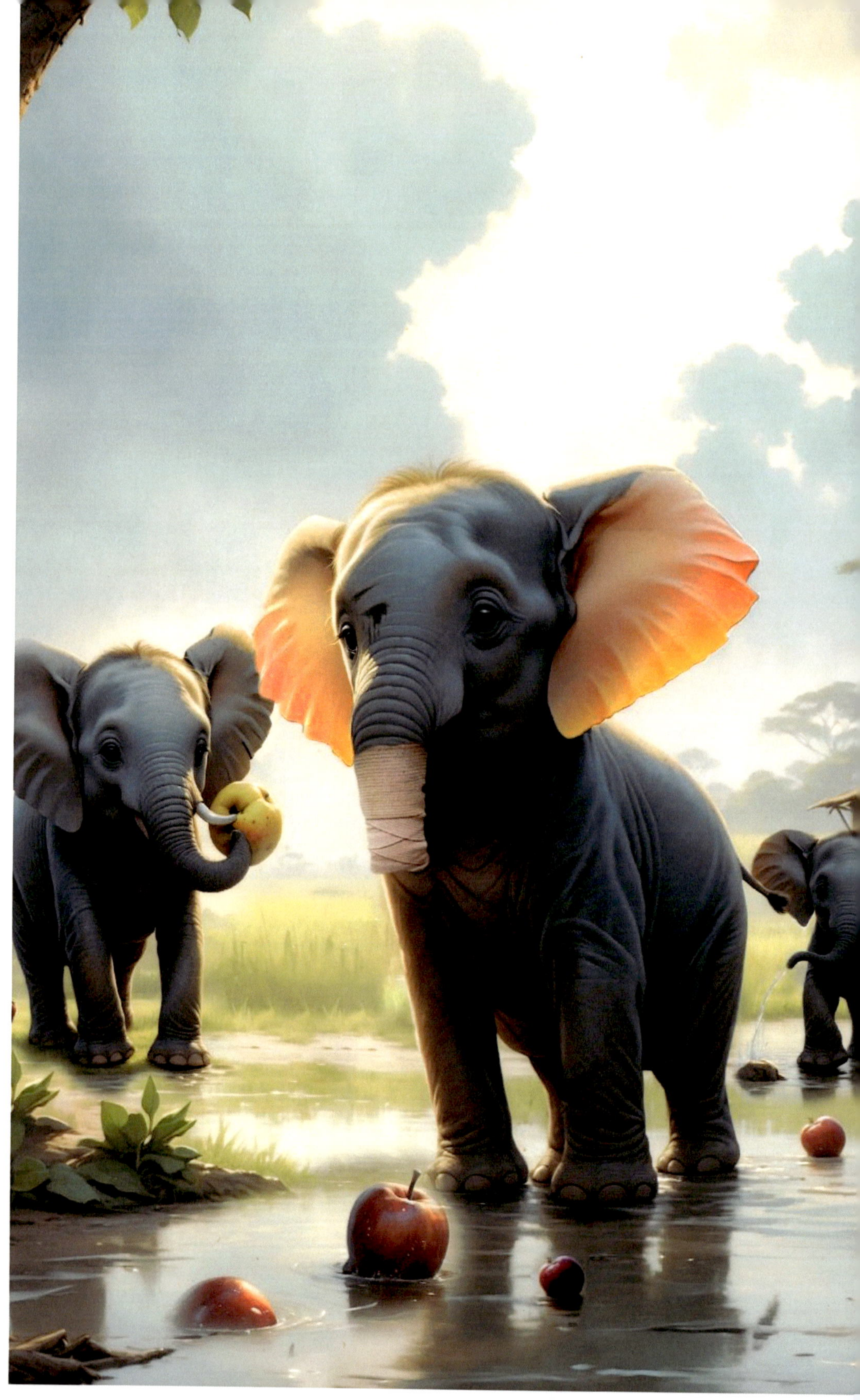

His friends were able to pluck fruits

from the trees and scoop water from the

rivers. Esinka hoped that he, too, could

find a way to eat and drink on his own.

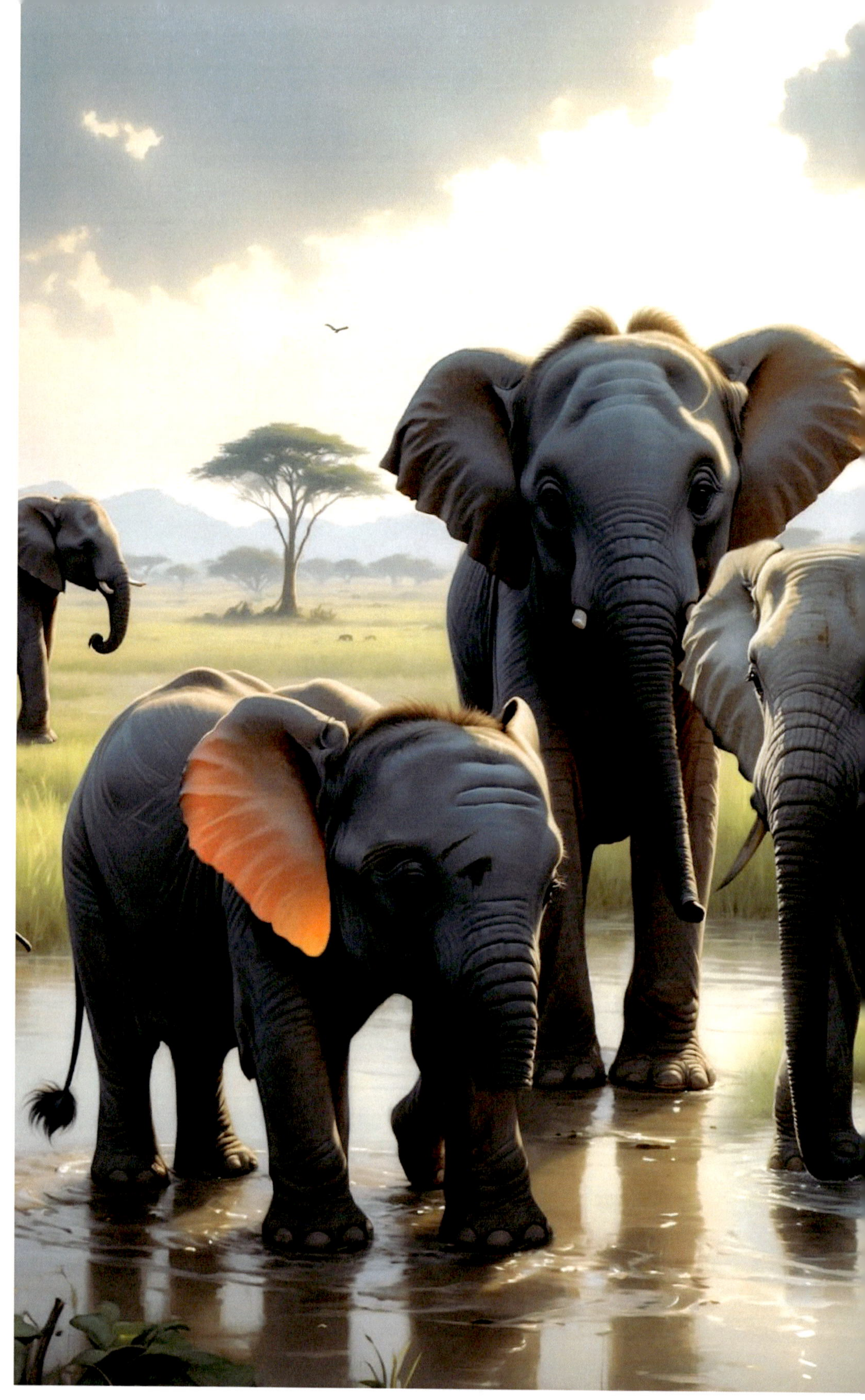

Drinking water, a simple thing for most

elephants, was very difficult for Esinka.

However, he refused to give up. Day

after day, he practiced bending down

and drinking water with only his short

trunk.

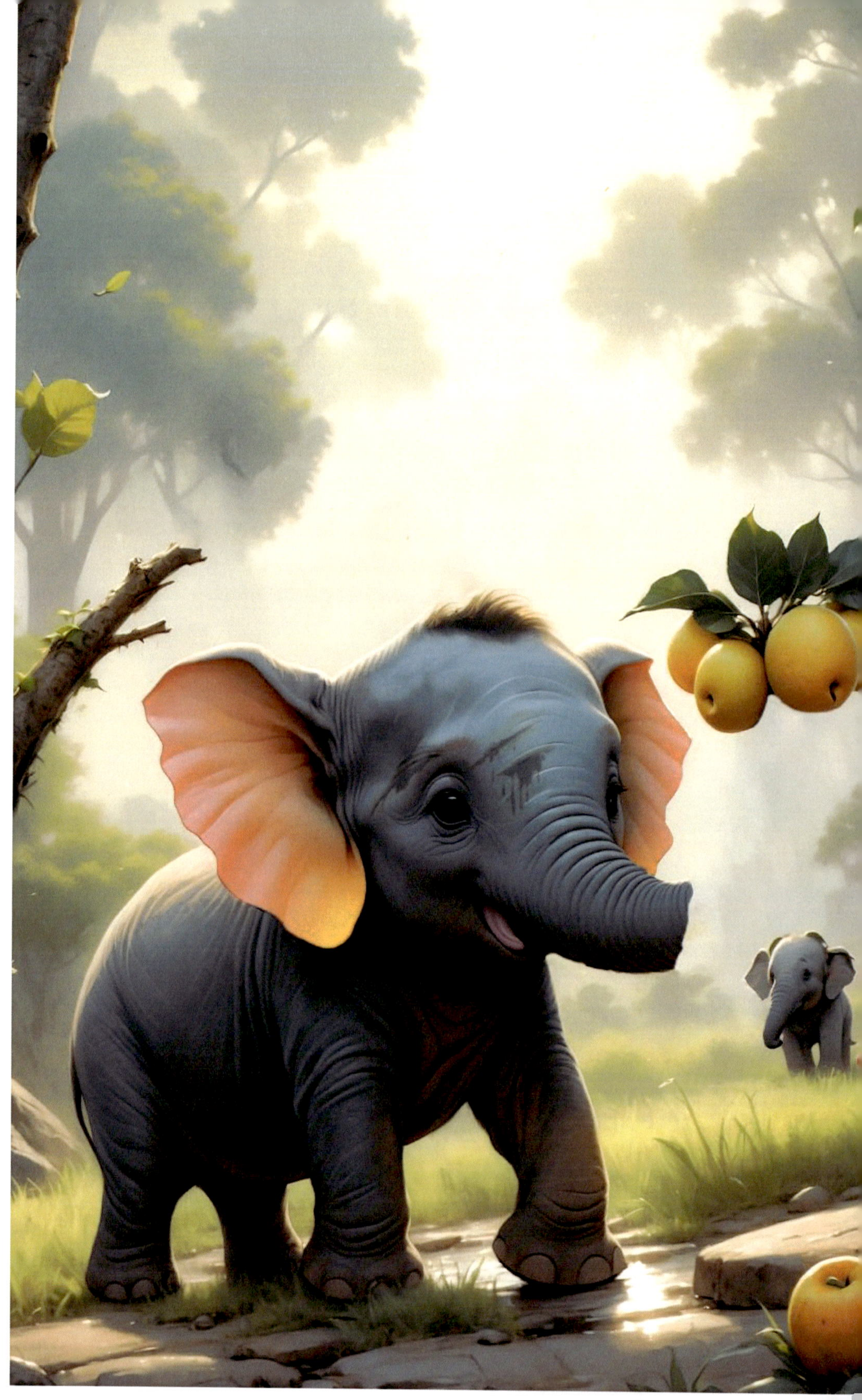

His friends also helped Esinka learn to use his trunk and his mouth to grab things. He learned to push fallen branches out of the way, pull himself up onto rocks, and grab leaves and fruit from the lower branches.

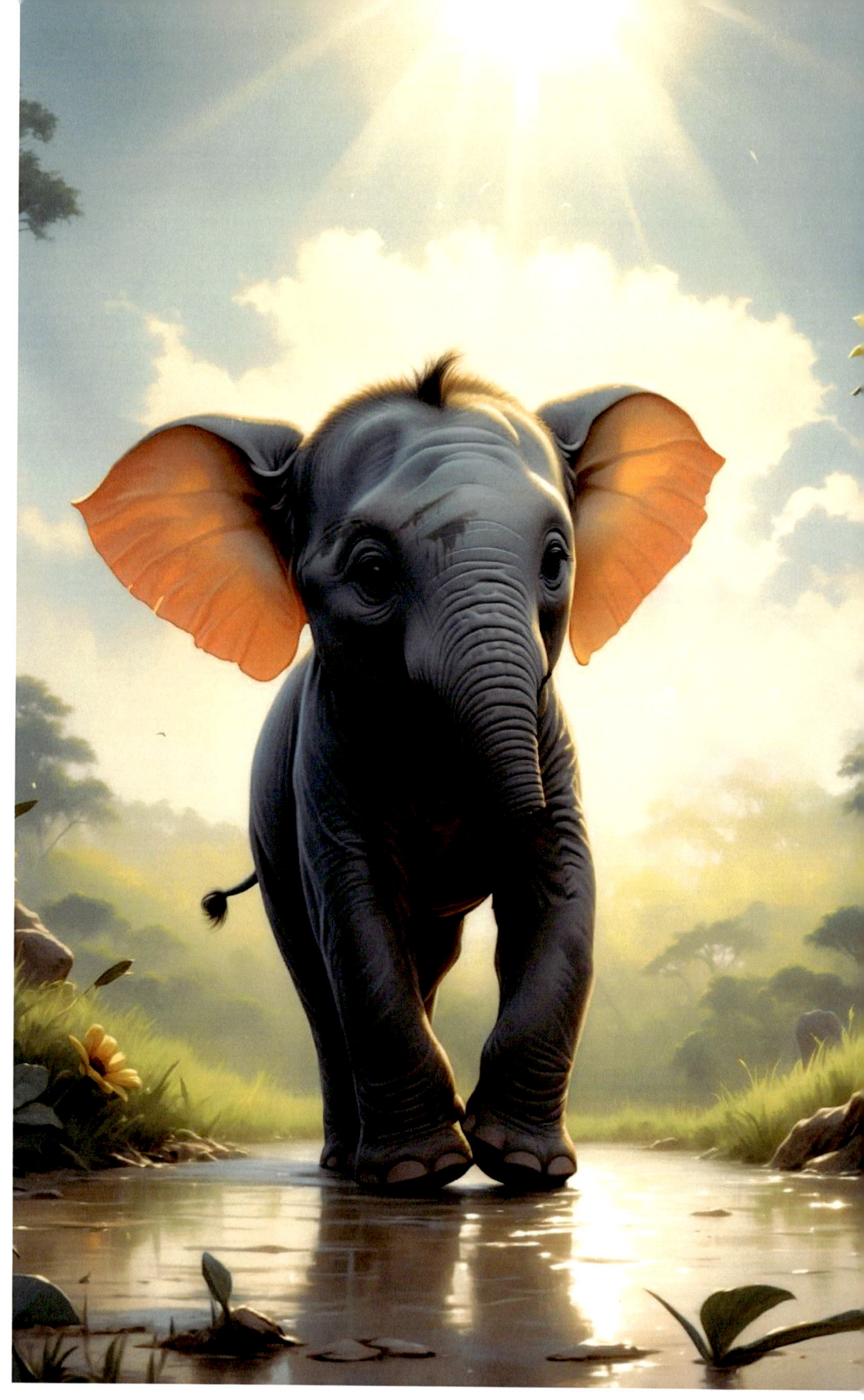

Even with many challenges, Esinka never lost sight of his dreams. With each passing day, he grew stronger and more confident, his courage shining bright like the African sun.

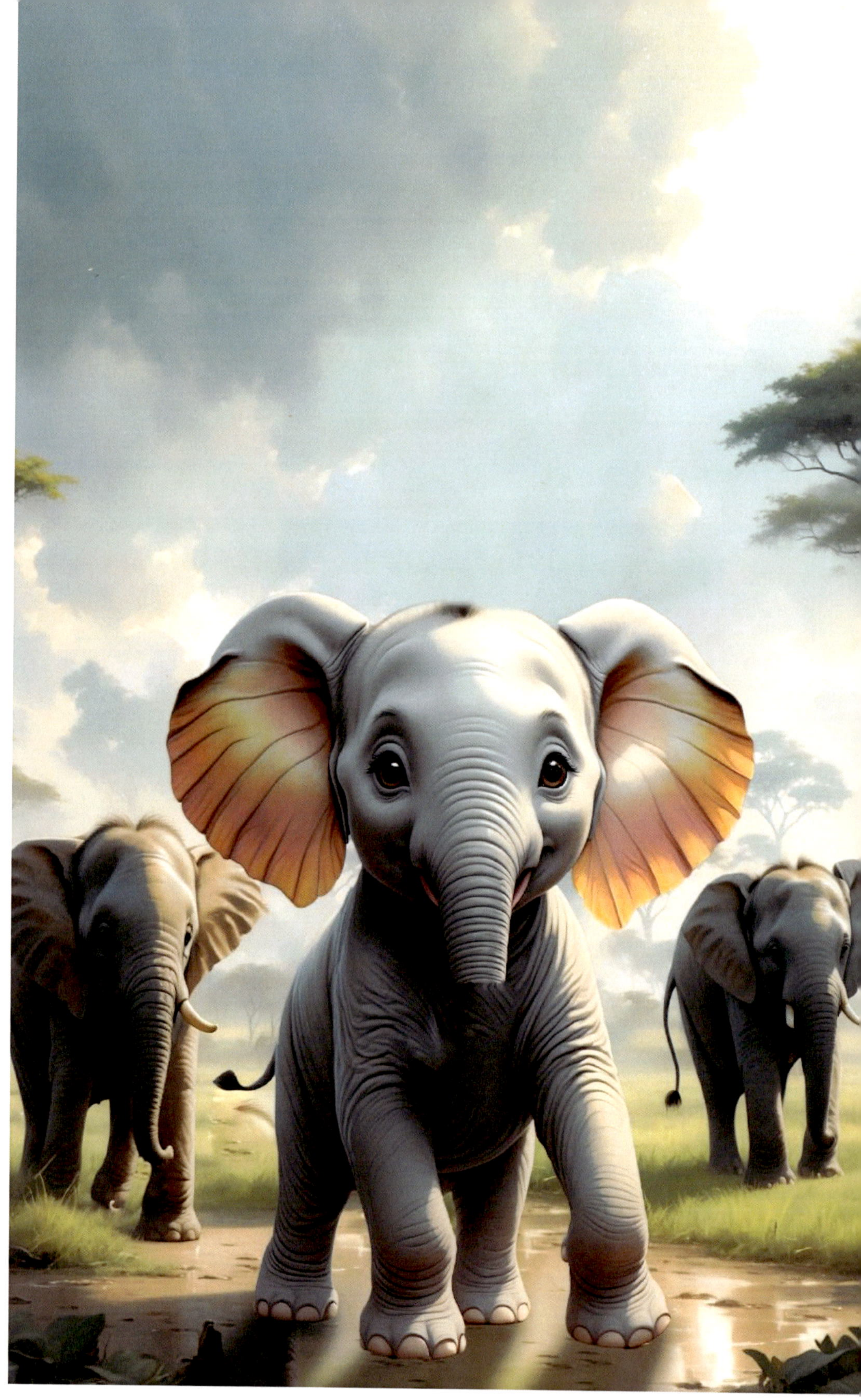

As the years went by, Esinka became

loved by all for his spirit and strength.

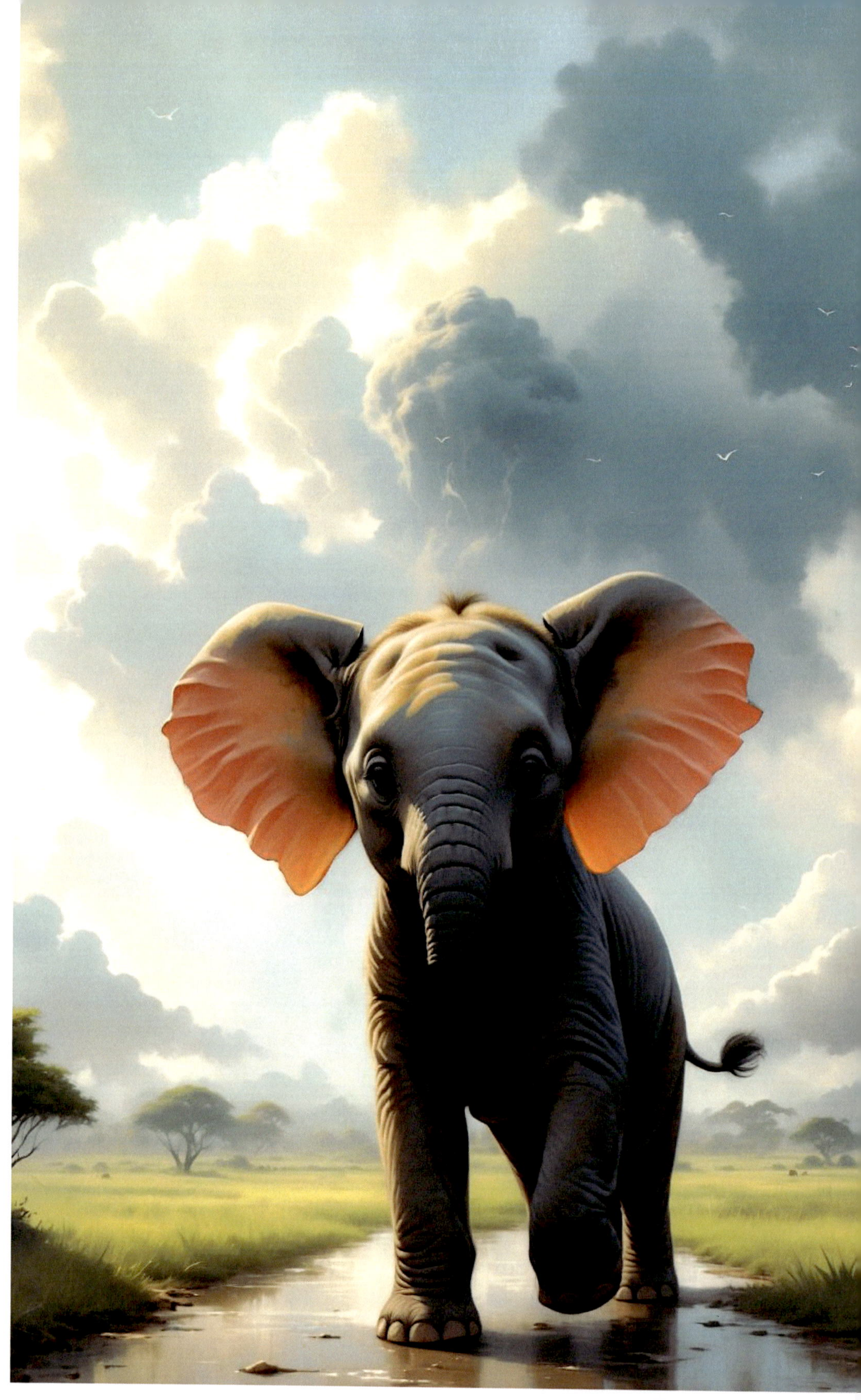

True courage, Esinka found out, was

not living in fear, but the willing to face

life with his new abilities.

Activity

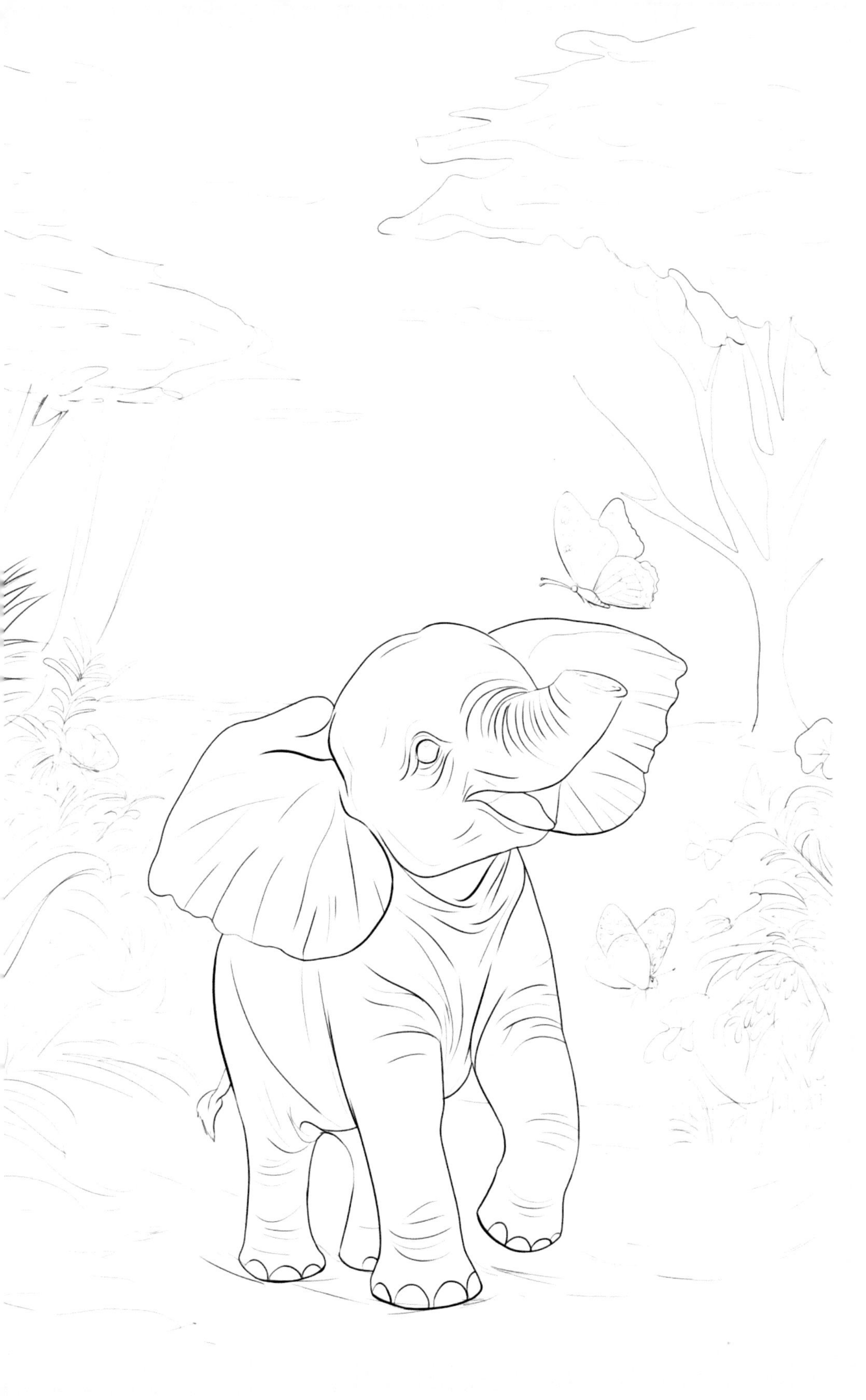

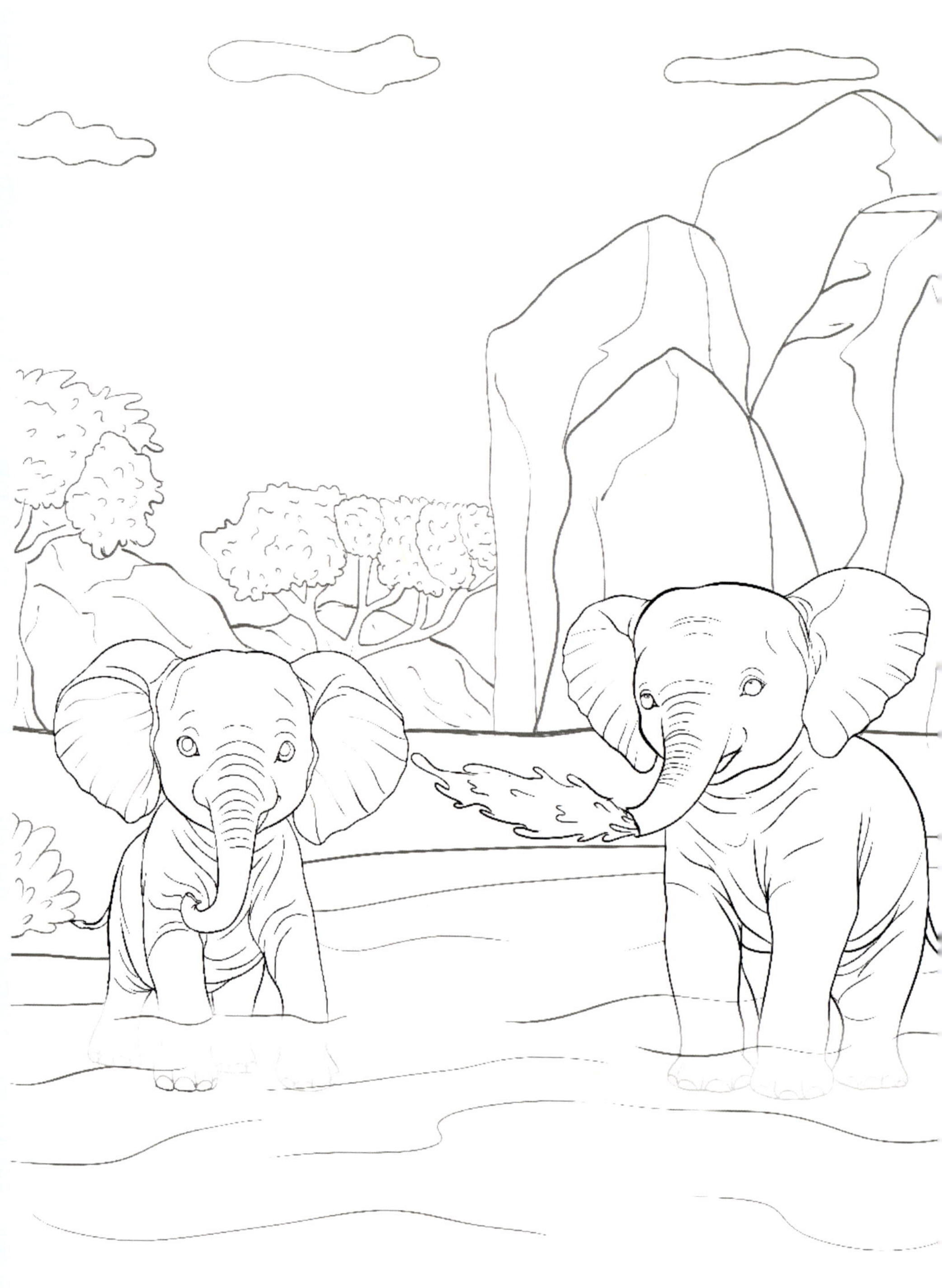

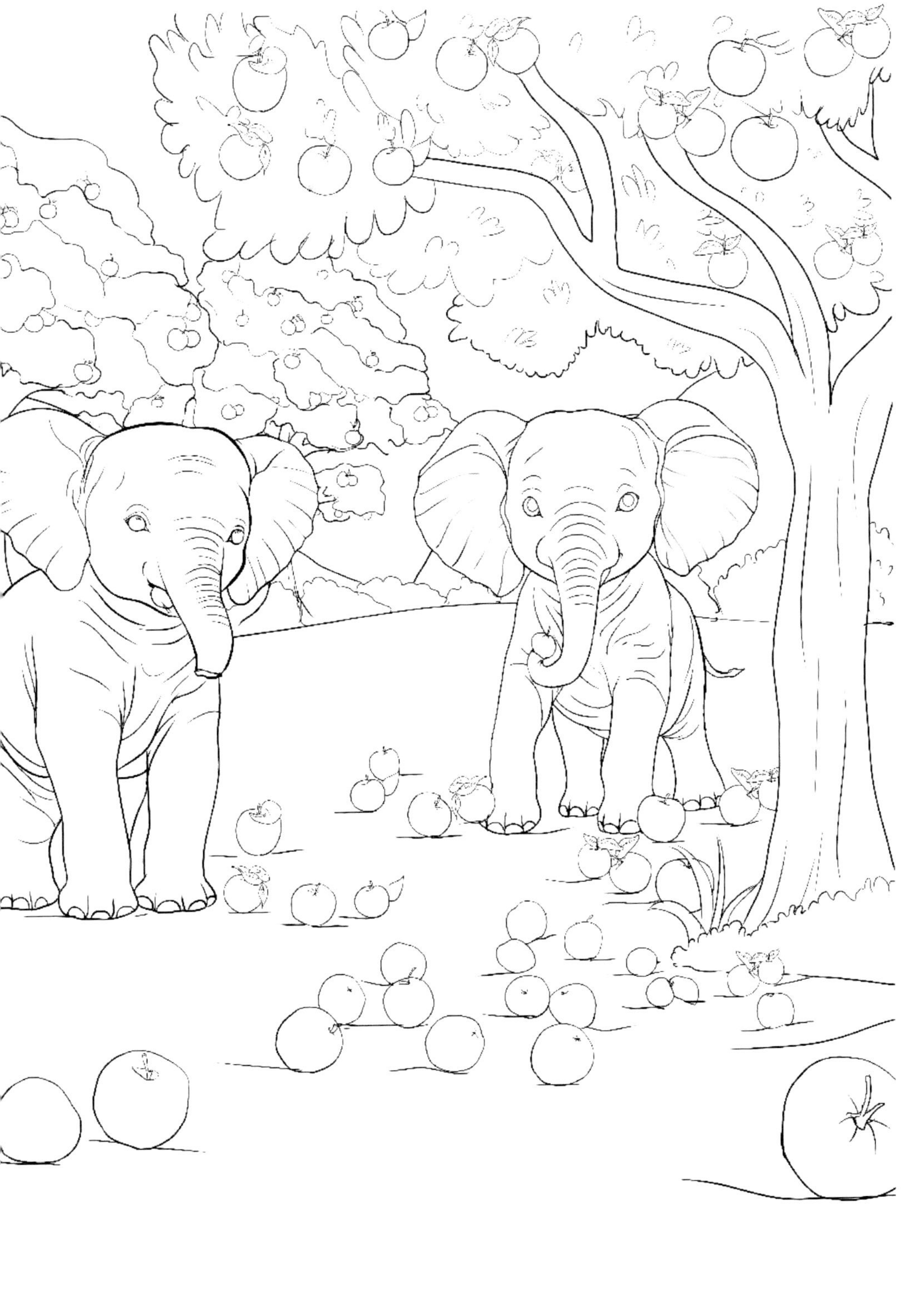

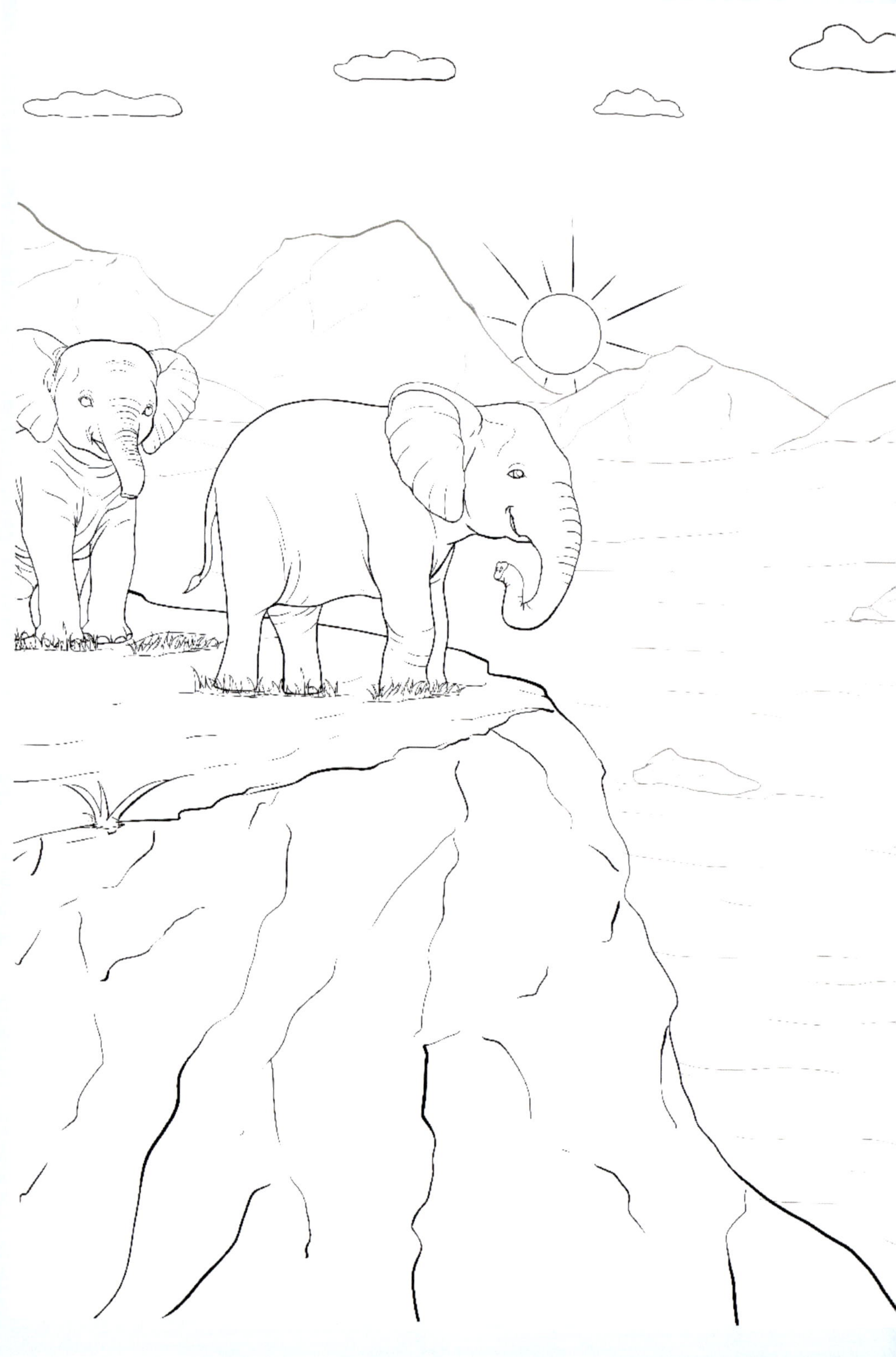

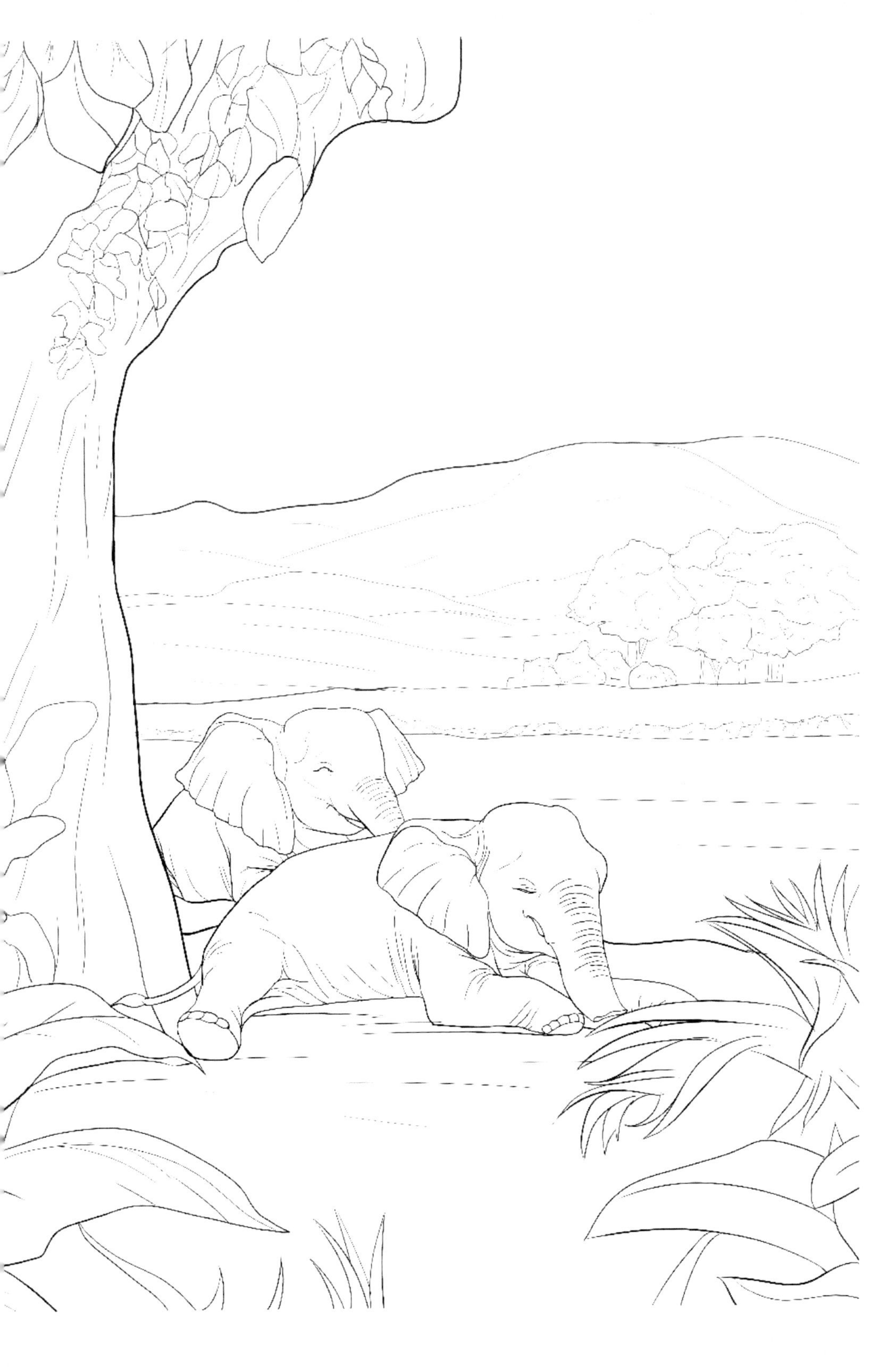

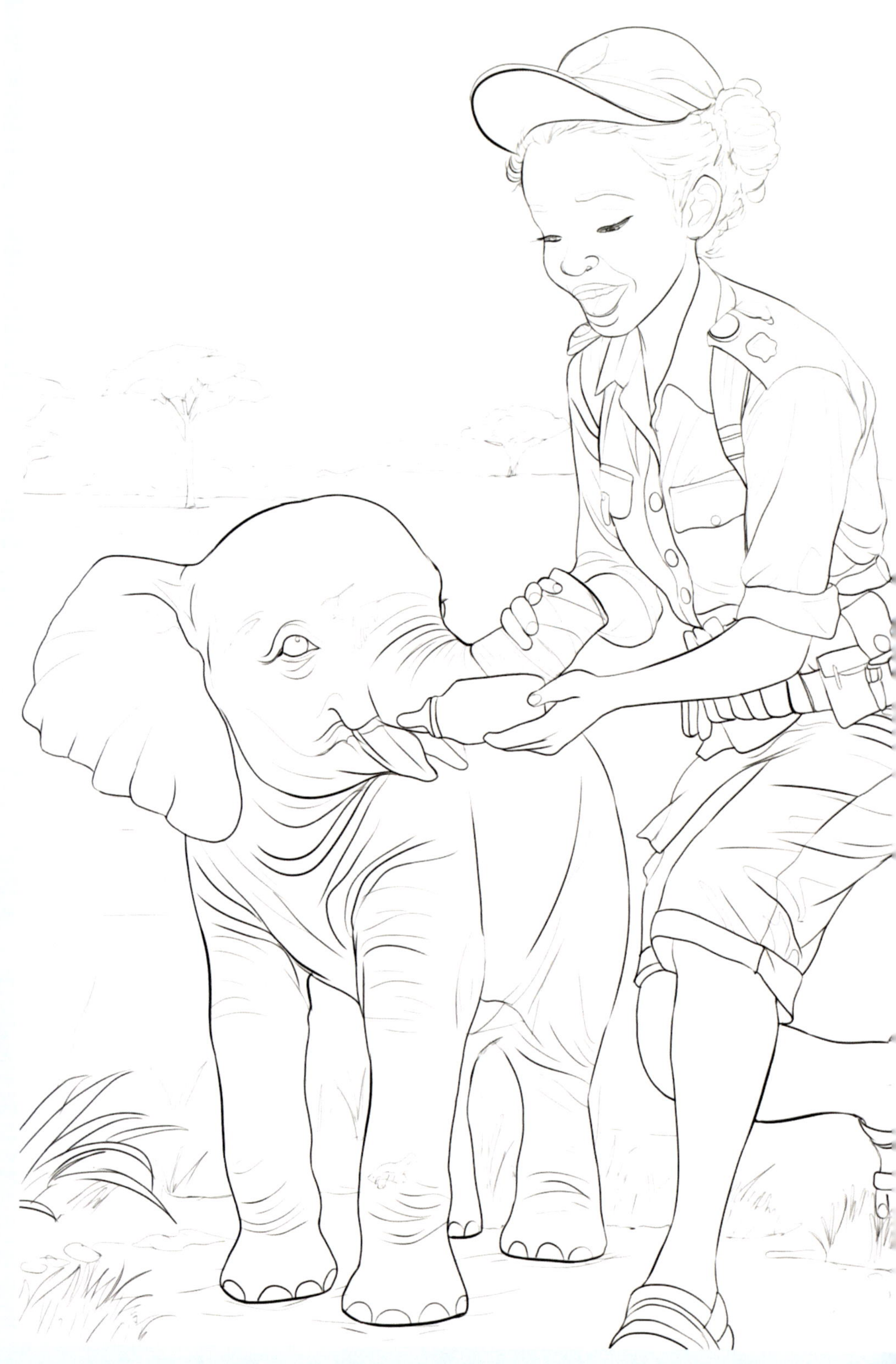